QUICK STEPS TO TAMING MS:
A CONCISE GUIDE TO MULTIPLE SCLEROSIS AND
IMMUNE SYSTEM REPAIR

by

Louise Docherty

Quick Steps to Taming MS: A Concise Guide to Multiple Sclerosis and Immune System Repair

Text and Cover Art ©2006 by Louise Docherty. All rights reserved.

No part of this book may be reproduced or transmitted in any form or by any means, electronic or mechanical, including photocopying or recording, or by any information storage and retrieval system, without written permission of Louise Docherty.

ORDER THIS BOOK at http://www.lulu.com

ISBN: 978-1-300-87175-0

CONTENTS

FOREWORD 5
MY MS STORY 9
WHAT IS MULTIPLE SCLEROSIS? 13
WHAT YOUR DOCTOR WILL DO 15
FIRST STEPS 17
BOOK NAVIGATION 19
GOODBYE TO GLUTEN 20
   Quick Guide to Sources of Gluten 21
   Gluten-Free Grains and Flours 23
KILL THE CANDIDA 24
   What exactly is Candida? 24
   What are the common symptoms of Candida? 24
   Why might you have Candida? 25
   How do you get rid of Candida? 26
      Things to Stop 26
      Things to Increase 26
OILS AND FATS 29
   Saturated Fats 29
   Essential Fatty Acids 29
      Linoleic Acid and Alpha-Linoleic Acid 29
      Evening Primrose Oil 31
      Hemp Oil 31
   Heated Oils Bad: Unheated Oils Good 32
      Hydrogenated Oils 32
   Hydrogenated Oil in Gluten-Free Products 33
   Storing Oils 34
VITAMINS AND MINERALS 35
   What to Take? 35
   Vitamin B_{12} 36
   Pycnogenol 37
   Vitamin D 37
   Eating Raw 38
   Coral Calcium 39
   Food Combining 39
BODY AND MIND 41
   Food Sensitivity Testing 41
   Physiotherapy 41

Exercise 41
  Qi Gong 42
  Visualization Techniques 42
  The MS Personality Profile 43
A TYPICAL DAY 44
  Morning 44
  Lunchtime 45
  Evening 45
SAMPLE MEAL PLANS 47
  SAMPLE MEAL PLAN: 1-12 WEEKS 49
  SAMPLE MEAL PLAN: 3-6 MONTHS 52
  SAMPLE MEAL PLAN: 6-12 MONTHS 55
YOUR CONTINUING HEALTH PLAN 58
A GET-STARTED-FAST BIBLIOGRAPHY 59

FOREWORD

It takes a long time for doctors to diagnose Multiple Sclerosis. In fact, the chances are you won't hear them use that term for quite a while. You are far more likely to hear them use the word *demyelination* and offer the advice *go home and rest*. But if you have demyelination (which is where the myelin sheath that protects the nerves in the Central Nervous System begins to break down), this is already a strong indication that you have MS, and you don't have time to wait until the doctors have confirmed it. If you have another attack (or 'episode', as your doctor is likely to call it), you are already far more likely to have another and another, and end up with relapsing-remitting MS, which eventually can reach a chronic state.

This is exactly the situation in which I found myself in the spring of 1998. The tests proved I had demyelination, but the diagnosis of MS was not possible. The only advice relevant to my particular situation was go home and rest. Which leads me to ask you this: are you a gambler?

I recently read in a medical dictionary that between 30-40% of people with MS-like symptoms will go into remission without lifestyle/diet changes or indeed medical intervention. In short, they do nothing. The dictionary goes on to add that this leaves sufferers of MS a prime target for dubious, alternative cures, where a patient may recover despite, and not because of, changes made in their lifestyle. But let's turn that statistic on its head, shall we? That means that between 60-70% of us *won't* go into remission by doing nothing. Now, I don't know about you, but I don't like those odds, and if making a few relatively simple lifestyle changes is going to change those odds in my favour, well, you can be damned sure I'm going to make them!

So, I went home and read everything on MS I could get my hands on. I made major lifestyle changes. I came to terms with the fact that MS is an autoimmune disease, imposed on me by the very defence system that is supposed to protect me. Yet, as an autoimmune disease, I believed it was ultimately under my control, if I could just figure out where I had gone wrong and how to get my body back.

Ultimately, I did. That MS 'episode' in 1998 is the one and only episode I have ever experienced. Whether that is a direct result of the changes I made in my diet and lifestyle can never be proven, but you can be sure of one thing: nothing I did caused me any harm. There are so many people who go home and do nothing, eventually succumbing to this degenerative disease. They allow their care to remain in the hands of their doctors. Their personal opportunity to act immediately is lost. They wait; and they suffer for it. In my opinion, doing nothing is the most dangerous thing you can do.

So there are two reasons why I wrote this book. The first is because I want you to do something *now*. The second is because I wanted to write the kind of book I wish I'd had when I was ill and exhausted, when sometimes picking up another 350-page book was the last thing I wanted to do. I wanted to write a guidebook; a quick book; if you like, a Coles Notes version of how to get your health back.

This is it. My Quick Steps book – with gratitude and acknowledgement to all those who put in the real hard graft and wrote the heavy books! With special thanks to all the people on the internet who are valiant enough to put their experiences online and give support to those who choose a route outside of the normal MS societies and doctors' waiting rooms.

And with special thanks to my husband, Patrick Docherty, who never hesitated to bring me home the heavy books in the first place and help me read them!

This Quick Steps summary is written for all the people over the last seven years who have asked me what I did and how I did it. This summary is also for you, a stranger, yet linked to all of us who live with this disease. Use it in good health!

MY MS STORY

March 1998. It started with the index finger of my left hand going numb and I didn't think much about it. After all, typing was a big part of how I made a living and we were always hearing about carpal tunnel syndrome. But three days later I woke up and the entire left side of my body, from the neck down, was numb.

I struggled on at work for a while, basically in denial. Whatever was wrong with me would go away. And if it didn't, it couldn't be that bad, could it? After all, my family doctor had said she would get me an appointment to see a neurologist and that appointment had arrived – it was for six months later. Not urgent, then.

People were worrying though. My parents were wondering if I'd had a stroke at the tender age of 36, or could it be something as simple as a trapped nerve? When I was doubled up in pain one night at work, I realised I could not ignore this any more. I took advantage of where I worked – a large law firm with access to our own specialist consultant in medical matters; a cardiologist, not a neurologist, but hey – my colleagues practically forced me into his office. I described my symptoms and he said he didn't think it was a stroke. He didn't say what he *did* think it was, but when he heard my appointment to see a neurologist was not for months, he got on the phone there and then and pulled a favour. I was in to see his neurologist buddy the day after the next.

Now, I was lucky. Because of a favour, I got to find out about demyelination (the doctors were still not using the MS word) months before I would have done otherwise, so I had months' head start. Even so, I was still in denial. It took a colleague at work, a veritable walking dictionary of a woman, to frown gently and say 'Demyelination? Hmm, you'd better hope you don't have that; that's not good.'

Not satisfied with the seven-month waiting list for an MRI under the Ontario health care system, my father paid for a private MRI scan in Buffalo, New York. The scan clearly showed the active areas of inflammation on the Central Nervous System – the mysterious demyelination! There was no denying it now. And yet I did. It was still only demyelination, not MS.

And then there came the morning I first experienced the symptom of banding around my chest – tight, numb strips that felt like ropes. I felt I couldn't breathe. I was beyond exhaustion. Another symptom of the illness. My husband phoned my neurologist, but the call was directed to his on-call colleague. At first, this doctor danced around what 'banding' might mean, but when my husband said the magic words – Multiple Sclerosis – the response was: 'Well, now that you've said it, we can talk about it.' Unbelievable, isn't it, that even the doctors skirt around a diagnosis of MS? No wonder I was in denial!

Again I was lucky. I phoned my work and told them the situation. I was put on short-term sick leave immediately. I was told to take as long as I needed. I think at that moment, not even being able to get out of bed, I finally realised it was up to me to take my health in hand. No one else was going to do it for me. No one else could.

Not being able to contemplate the thought of even the simplest meal preparation, and with my husband not being able to take any time off work to look after me, we took me over to my wonderful mother-in-law's, and nearly every night my husband would come over and we would discuss my recovery plan. He invariably came laden with books, vitamins, or some other health potion he'd managed to find out about. I tried to read everything I could, while putting into practice the bits and pieces that seemed to make the most sense to me. Number one: cut out gluten. Number two: attack Candida. Number three: exercise. Number four: deep breathe, visualize. Every day I dragged myself around the block, my mother-in-law Jackie at my side, my feet like blocks of wood. My gait changed. I lost motor skills in my arms, hands and legs. At night I kept hitting myself in the face with my left hand, having no idea where the limb in fact was.

There was pain too. Pain in my joints, pain in my muscles. I had a hard time getting my head around the fact that this pain didn't really exist where I thought it did. It might have felt like I had pain in my fingers, but the problem really lay in the inflammation on the Central Nervous System, specifically in my neck. My brain and my body weren't communicating properly, and boy did I know about it!

But slowly there came an improvement. Every morning I would wake up and try and guess where my left hand was. At first I was always 100% wrong. After two weeks, I felt I *almost* knew where it was. Suddenly, at three weeks, I got it right! And the banding started to reduce, the numbness moving down and away from my chest. At the same time, my legs started to come back to me; my arms followed. The numbness seemed to be always moving down, away from me, away from my brain, leaving my body out through my feet. I remembered my Chinese acupuncturist saying once that pain moving down was a good thing, so this had to be good. I persisted with my health routine. I increased my walking time. At the end of the third week I went back home.

A week later I had an appointment with my neurologist. 'Whatever you're doing,' he said, 'you're months ahead in recovery.' I started to tell him, but he raised his hand and shook his head. 'Don't,' he said. 'It's not that I won't believe you, it's just that I can't tell my other patients what you're doing. It's not medically proven.' I have always thought what a strange, sad state of affairs this was – this obviously caring and dedicated professional bound by a medical convention that refuses to discuss anecdotal evidence to the extent of saying nothing. What harm could it do, I thought, to tell someone not to eat gluten? I guess his answer would have been, 'What is my liability, if I tell someone not to eat gluten and they get worse?' I understand that position, but I think, you doctors of medicine, that you do us, your patients, a great disservice. Let me have all the information, no matter how 'off the wall'. Tell me there's no scientific proof, but let *me* decide!

It's now 2006. I have never had a second attack and I am told to go five years without a second episode puts me into the 'benign MS' category. If you're reading this book and you're having an episode, you can rest assured I know exactly what you're going through. If you are having optic disturbances and dizziness, I appreciate that that will make reading and movement harder for you, but you must concentrate *right now* on finding your way back to good health and managing MS through diet and exercise, body and mind. The sooner you do it, the more likely it will be that you avoid the worst ravages of this degenerative disease. If you ever feel unmotivated, ask yourself the one question I asked myself every time I was tempted to cheat: do you want to end up in a wheelchair?

I would hope no one's going to say yes to that!

WHAT IS MULTIPLE SCLEROSIS?

Multiple Sclerosis manifests itself in several ways: numbness, tingling, loss of balance, loss of bladder control, vision impairment, loss of dexterity, loss of motor-coordination, banding (a sensation of tightness across the trunk), unexplained pain in joints and muscles, and extreme fatigue. The symptoms are caused by an autoimmune response where the body attacks the myelin sheath that surrounds the nerves in the Central Nervous System (CNS). This process is called *demyelination*, and causes disruption of signals between the brain and the body – just like an exposed electrical wire. Eventually, the myelin sheath repairs itself, but often scarring remains ('sclerosis'), which continues to impair CNS function. When there are multiple scars, it is known as 'multiple sclerosis'.

The medical community still doesn't know what causes the immune system to attack the CNS, causing these multiple scars. One of the theories is that it's caused by the Herpes 6 virus, a very common virus that in most people is harmless. Another is that it's something to do with hormones. Another, lack of Vitamin D. Scientific attention is focused on developing a drug to suppress the MS sufferer's over-active immune system - to stop the body attacking itself. This is a reactive response, one of 'if your immune system does this, we will do this.' We, on the other hand, are not going to wait for further symptoms: we are going to repair our immune system and hence the root cause. We are going to be proactive.

There are several types of MS:

(1) single episodes, where a person might experience one attack during their lifetime, or go many, many years between episodes, which do not worsen in severity (benign MS);
(2) relapsing/remitting MS (the most common), where the episodes occur fairly frequently (every 1-2 years) and do not worsen; and
(3) chronic MS, where relapsing/remitting develops into an ongoing, worsening condition.

So far the medical community's response to MS varies from 'go home and rest' to implementing a course of steroids (which provides short-term relief from inflammation on the CNS) and, most recently, beta-interferon drugs. These latter drugs have been shown to greatly relieve symptoms, but in some cases the side-effects have created serious problems (particularly liver damage). Yet, despite all this, the medical community cannot tell us what causes MS and research continues to be focused on finding the perfect drug to combat the symptoms.

The approach I took was to treat the whole immune system, not just the symptoms.

WHAT YOUR DOCTOR WILL DO

Your GP may first do blood tests. He'll be looking for Vitamin B_{12} deficiency, which can lead to neurological disorders. My result came back normal. Your GP will then refer you to a neurologist.

You may wait months to see this neurologist, unless you're lucky. He will check you out and give you a number of simple tests, such as holding your arms out straight in front of you with your eyes closed to see if you can hold them at an equal height. This tests the fine sensors of your nerve endings. You will also be given dexterity tests, balance tests and vision tests.

You will probably be sent for something called Evoked Response Testing, where the electrical impulses between the brain and the nerves are tested and measured for deterioration. You may even be sent for an MRI. An MRI (Magnetic Resonance Imaging) is one of the surest ways to confirm demyelination, as any areas of active inflammation on the CNS will show up on the MRI scan. However, not everyone gets one of these expensive scans, and those of us who get one may wait months for the privilege, unless you are able to pay for it yourself.

You get the picture – TIME IS GOING ON!

No matter how sympathetic and professional your GP and neurologist are, both of them are bound by the conventions of scientific medicine to send you for tests that will take weeks, if not months, to complete. (And even so, I was told I wouldn't get a diagnosis of MS until I'd had another attack.) In the meantime, they will tell you to go home and rest. They might prescribe steroids, often used when there are vision disturbances and bladder problems. Thankfully, I was never bad enough to consider the use of steroids, and personally I would have resisted taking them, since, in my opinion, these only treat the symptoms of MS, not the underlying cause, and come with a whole range of side-effects themselves. Moreover, I believe they may undermine your own ability to tell the true state of your health by screening out your symptoms. If you do find yourself on steroids due to the severity of your symptoms, don't forget that you still have a serious, degenerative illness and you have to nip it in the bud as soon as possible by concentrating on repairing your immune system. Steroids will not do that for you.

Immune system dysfunction requires active intervention NOW! Do not go home and do nothing. Go home and embark upon repairing your health!

FIRST STEPS

Let's assume the best-case scenario.

- You are able to take a hefty chunk of sick leave and not worry about bills
- You have a supportive partner or family
- You have money to buy vitamins and health foods
- You have access to alternative healthcare practitioners, such as naturopaths
- You have willpower

Now let's look at the opposite.

- You can't get paid sick leave
- Your family don't understand how MS makes you feel and expect you to carry on pretty much as normal
- Your budget isn't going to stretch to fancy vitamins and organic foods
- What's a naturopath and where do you find one
- You just aren't selfish enough to put yourself first

Take heart. Whatever your circumstances, you can do a lot, even if you find yourself in a not particularly supportive environment. That's because the changes you desire ultimately come from within you, and are not necessarily dependent on external factors. (After all, you can be wealthy and single and still get MS!) The number one thing is making sure that you and your loved ones understand one simple thing: putting yourself first is not selfish. Putting yourself first ensures your best health scenario, which ultimately benefits everyone.

Above I've outlined the best and worst case scenarios. Below I outline important steps to improving your health. The assumption is that you will have circumstances that are closer to the best case scenario than the worst case scenario. If this is not your situation, you may need to rely on outside resources. Check for support groups for MS or other autoimmune disorders in your area if you find your circumstances lead towards the worst case scenario.

Therefore, Step 1 is your *self*. Make a decision to make yourself a priority. If you have young children or other dependents, it's going to be down to your partner or family to carry most of the load, because if you are having an MS episode you are probably exhausted.

Step 2: open your mind. There are a lot of things out there that are going to help you get better, and doctors are involved in very few of them.

Step 3: be prepared to change on a mental level. You didn't get MS just from eating badly, or having a genetic predisposition, or catching a retro-virus, or whatever new medical research suggests is a factor causing MS. There was another piece of the puzzle: you. How you react to the world, particularly stress, is a contributing factor.

Step 4: be prepared to spend the money. The way back to good health doesn't have to be expensive, but if you have any spare cash, spend it first on *health*.

Step 5: give it time. You didn't get ill overnight; why expect to be better overnight? Your body is trying to rebalance itself, so stick with it and give it time to do its job.

BOOK NAVIGATION

The following sections in this book are divided into the changes you are going to make in your life in order to maximize your chances for recovery. Simply, they will discuss:

Gluten
Candida
Fats and Oils
Vitamins and Supplements
Body and Mind
A Typical Day
Sample Meal Plans

Each section is designed to get you started quickly. Remember, this book is designed for people who might have very little energy to spare right now. For more in-depth research, you can consult the bibliography, or indeed conduct your own searches in bookstores and on the Internet. There is always new information coming out on MS and I am the first to admit I am not educated in all of it.

Now let's move on to all the things you are going to do to rebuild your health!

GOODBYE TO GLUTEN

If there was one thing that I believe led to an almost instant improvement in my symptoms of numbness, banding and dexterity, it was cutting out *gluten*.

Gluten is the protein found in *wheat, rye*, and *barley*, and to a lesser degree in *spelt* and *kamut*. It is also debatable whether gluten is in *oats*. Some believe it is only present in oats due to cross-contamination with wheat at food processing centres, and there has been recent research carried out in the U.S. that suggests oats can be safely eaten in a gluten-free diet. However, at the time I was making my diet changes, I stopped eating oats for a year (instead eating millet, rice and quinoa cereals), and introduced oats back into my diet when I was feeling much better. I continue to eat oats today, and indeed there seems to be more research all the time that supports the argument that oats belong to a different group of cereals than wheat, rye and barley, containing both a protein different in structure and in quantity. If you want to do what I did, cut them out for now. You can always add them back in later.

The official name for someone who is gluten intolerant is a *celiac*. Now, you might not be a celiac, and personally I have never been tested for gluten-intolerance (celiac disease can be tested for with blood tests, but only definitely proven with a small bowel biopsy.) However, so many people on the MS websites were talking about the improvements in their neurological symptoms after eliminating gluten from their diets that it seemed insane not to try it. I was not disappointed. Within three weeks of cutting out gluten, the banding around my trunk had almost disappeared, I had regained the ability to know where my left hand was when I closed my eyes, and the numbness in my legs, trunk, back and arms had greatly reduced. Perhaps this was due to a combination of all the other life-style changes I was making, but I feel the elimination of gluten brought about the quickest and most apparent improvement.

So what does cutting out gluten involve? Well, it's goodbye to bread, pasta, pastry and anything that contains flour. That includes cakes and biscuits, gravies and soups containing flour, stock cubes containing flour – would you believe that even some ground spices contain flour (they use it to stop the spices clumping together)? Read labels like your life depends on it. And don't rely on health store staff regarding gluten advice – I have been told in the past that kamut and spelt are gluten-free. Wrong. They are *wheat* free. Big difference.

When I cut out gluten it was still not generally known what gluten was. I am pleased to say that you can now go in a restaurant and stand a good chance of your waiter knowing exactly what gluten is and how to go about giving you something off the menu that you can eat. Perhaps this is not too surprising – I read recently that they now think over 50% of the population of North America is gluten-sensitive. That's not the same as being celiac, but it's a big enough statistic that it's got the food industry's attention. You can see the evidence of that in all the new gluten-free products that are on the shelves. However, a quick read of the labels on these products reveals a host of harmful ingredients, so beware! More on these tempting treats and their doubtful benefits later! (See the section Hydrogenated Oil in Gluten-Free Products, below.)

No one has proved the link between gluten and MS, as your neurologist will remind you. You might not even be a celiac. All this is irrelevant. Your goal is to reach a state of health where you will not experience any relapse. If people who have MS are saying they feel better by not eating gluten, then *stop eating it!* It might be one of the hardest things you will have to give up, but I say if it comes to a choice between eating a piece of toast and having a relapse, there's just no contest.

Quick Guide to Sources of Gluten

Definitely contains gluten:
- Baking powder (contains wheat)
- Barley
- Bulgar
- Couscous
- Kamut

- Malt (made from barley)
- Malt vinegar
- Pasta of any kind (contains durum wheat flour)
- Rye
- Sausages (contain breadcrumbs/rusk)
- Semolina
- Soy Sauce (contains wheat)
- Spelt
- Veggie dogs (contain flour)
- Wheat

- and any products made of the above, such as:
    - Biscuits
    - Breads
    - Buns
    - Cakes
    - Pastry
    - Croutons
    - Crisp breads

Possible sources of gluten:
- Blue Cheese (can contain wheat, which makes the mould)
- Burgers (may contain bread crumbs)
- Dried fruits (some may contain flour to stop them sticking together)
- Oats (as discussed above, may or may not. Cut out for now to be safe.)
- Sauces (may contain wheat flour as a thickener)
- Some ground herbs and spices (mixed with flour to stop them clumping together in the bottle). To be safe, grind your own (a coffee grinder is good for this).
- Soups (may contain wheat flour as a thickener)

Hidden sources of gluten:
- Anything brewed with hops or malt (e.g. beer, scotch)
- HVP (hydrolysed vegetable protein) – made from wheat

- MSG (monosodium glutamate). Avoid this like the plague. Usually found in store-bought stock cubes, soups, flavoured crisps and nuts, and ready meals. Its E-number is E621.
- Rice milk and soya milk drinks (often made using a barley process. To be on the safe side I never drink these.)
- Starch – may be made from wheat. Cornstarch is fine.

Above all, be very careful reading labels. Don't read the marketing label; read the ingredients label. Corn muffins might lead you to think they're made only of corn, but they probably also contain wheat flour. If there is no label, ask. If no one knows the answer, don't buy it.

Gluten-Free Grains and Flours

- Amaranth
- Arrowroot
- Buckwheat
- Cassava
- Chickpea
- Corn
- Cream of Tartar and Bicarbonate of Soda (combine together to make your own gluten-free Baking Powder)
- Flax seed
- Lentil
- Millet
- Potato
- Quinoa
- Rice
- Soya
- Tapioca
- Wild rice (actually a grass)

KILL THE CANDIDA

There are dozens of books on Candida, and in this section I am going to attempt to give you the basics, bearing in mind the goal of this handbook – to provide people who are ill with a quick and easy path to help them get started on the road back to health. For anyone who wants to know more about Candida, there is plenty of reading material out there, some of which I list in the bibliography.

What exactly is Candida?

Candida is an overgrowth of yeast in the gut. It is bad bacteria. If you imagine that your gut is a perfectly balanced garden of healthy intestinal flora, Candida is the weeds run amok. Candida is in all of us – the problem arises when it gets out of control. It takes food away from the good bacteria that keep our immune system healthy; it steals nourishment from the body; it prevents proper absorption of vitamins and minerals; and it leaves us a sitting duck for other, more deadly viruses, bacteria and parasites. Most worryingly, one school of thought believes Candida has the power to breach the blood-brain barrier, which can cause autoimmune dysfunction (seen in degenerative diseases such as Alzheimer's, Multiple Sclerosis, Rheumatoid Arthritis, and Lou Gehrig's Disease).

You can obviously see the relevance in regard to MS: Candida interferes with our immune system and might even impair the CNS (Central Nervous System).

What are the common symptoms of Candida?

The following is a list of symptoms:

- Diarrhoea
- Constipation
- Bloating
- Excessive flatulence
- Heartburn
- Depression
- Irritability
- Lack of concentration
- Acne
- Cystitis
- Menstrual problems
- Thrush (yeast infections)

- Hopelessness
- Anxiety
- Migraine
- Fatigue

Plus all the illnesses that Candida stops our immune system from fighting, such as colds, flu, gastric upsets, and general susceptibility to viral infections.

Candida has also been associated with the neurological problems of tingling and numbness in the limbs.

Why might you have Candida?

Lots of things can encourage a yeast overgrowth in your gut, but they are all to do with things you ingest, so remember that ultimately you have power over them.

You might have Candida from eating too much of the wrong foods. Candida loves sugar in all its forms (*i.e.* refined sugar, brown sugar, honey, molasses, corn syrup, dextrose, even fruit sugar). It loves dairy products – milk products contain their own form of sugar (lactose), as well as being generally hard to digest, which allows the Candida bad bacteria to stick around in the gut and cause your partially digested food to rot. It loves mouldy foods e.g. cheese, mushrooms, peanuts, cashews and dried fruits. It loves alcohol and similarly grapes and vinegar. It simply adores yeast, which is of course in most of our breads. And also it loves refined products such as white flour, white rice and pasta, because these foods have had most of their nutrients removed and will not feed the good bacteria in your gut, which ultimately would drive back the Candida to a more healthy level.

You might also have Candida if you've ever been on a long course of antibiotics, or have used the birth control pill. Such drugs wipe out your good intestinal flora and allow Candida to go on the rampage.

How do you get rid of Candida?

This is the good news: *you* can get rid of Candida. It just takes time. As you successfully reduce the Candida in your body, you might experience a symptom called 'die-off', where you feel blocked up, stuffy, as if you are coming down with a cold or flu. Don't let this deter you.

Things to Stop

- Cut out sugar in all its forms. For the first 6 weeks this also includes all fruit, as you are trying to starve out the Candida, and even the fruit sugar will allow the Candida to hang on. The exception to this is fresh pineapple (not tinned), as pineapple contains enzymes that act as a wonderful digestive. (Note: if you are fortunate enough to be able to find a naturopath who will give you food sensitivity testing, you might be advised that it is all right for you to eat various fruits. I would still recommend against it for 5-6 weeks. Once your Candida has dropped, you can reintroduce fruit in small quantities.)

- Cut out milk, cheese, mushrooms, peanuts, cashews, dried fruits, alcohol, vinegar, yeast and white rice.

- Cut out caffeine and don't use tea bags (which can harbour mould).

- Reduce your consumption of meat and poultry, both of which take a long time to digest and sit around in the gut fermenting and encouraging bad bacteria and parasites. I kept a small amount of chicken in my diet, cutting out red meat altogether.

Things to Increase

- Increase your intake of foods that kill Candida and parasites. The ones I know of are garlic, ginger, cumin, turmeric, coriander, cayenne pepper, pumpkin seeds and taheebo tea (also known as Pau D'Arco), which is made from the bark of the taheebo tree in the Amazon.

- Eat brown rice, not white.

- Eat low-fat yoghurt (the only exception to the dairy blacklist), preferably goat's milk or sheep's milk yoghurt, which is more easily digested than cow's milk. Make sure it is natural yoghurt containing *live* bacteria with *no* sugar or honey. The label usually tells you whether it contains live bacteria (don't assume all yoghurt does).

- I also went on supplements of *Acidophilus* (the bacteria found in yoghurt) in order to increase the helpful bacteria in the gut. If you are intolerant of dairy products, you should make sure you buy your Acidophilus in a non-dairy base. The health store people will be able to advise you on this.

- Get at least ½ hour of natural daylight on your eyes each day (no eyeglasses, no contact lenses). Natural light kills Candida.

A naturopath is a great asset in helping you get rid of Candida, but that may be a cost you can't afford. If so, may I suggest that you spend the money instead on Acidophilus and also on anything containing Black Walnut, Wormwood, Clove Oil, and Grapefruit Seed Extract. There are many combinations of this, but basically you are looking for an anti-parasitical/anti-Candida remedy, either in capsule or drop form. Again, a good health shop can help you find a product. Below is the regimen that I personally followed:

- On waking, drink a glass or two of boiled warm or hot water with a slice of lemon in it (a cleanser for the body). Do not eat anything for ½ hr-1 hr.

- After every meal, wait 10 minutes, then take your Black Walnut capsule or drops (or equivalent anti-parasitical). Wait another 10 minutes, then take your Acidophilus capsule. (Do this routine rather than what might be recommended on the bottle instructions.) Follow this routine 3 times a day for at least 6 weeks. What you are doing is killing the bad bacteria, then replenishing your gut with good bacteria. This should really bring down the Candida.

OILS AND FATS

The correct intake of oils and fats is crucial to MS sufferers, seeing that the myelin sheath is made up mainly of lipids i.e. complex fats. Most of what I did (and continue to do) in my own healing process is attributable to the advice given by Udo Erasmus in his book *Fats that Heal, Fats that Kill*, the advice given by Judy Graham in her book *Multiple Sclerosis – A Self-Help Guide To Its Management* (particularly the advice relating to Evening Primrose Oil), and to the advice given by Dr R Swank following his studies on the effects of oils and fats on MS patients. What follows below is the barest summary of the health advantages of oils and fats discussed in the books I have just mentioned. Again, I am adhering to the goal of this MS Handbook – to tell you what I did and to get you started quickly!

Saturated Fats

Decrease your intake of saturated fats. This is good for everyone, but one of the few areas where the medical community agrees is that people with MS have a problem handling saturated fat. Dr R Swank (the Swank Diet) recommends not more than 15 grams of saturated fat per day for the MS sufferer. If you consider that the average American ingests 40 grams of saturated fat per day, you can appreciate the difference. Be careful reading food labels, though. Most of them just give the total fat content i.e. fats coming from saturated *and* essential fatty acids. Also be aware that when sugar is absorbed into the body, it turns into saturated fat. (However, if you are being good and following the anti-Candida recommendations, you should not be ingesting many sugar sources!)

Essential Fatty Acids

Linoleic Acid and Alpha-Linoleic Acid

Essential Fatty Acids (EFAs) fall into two main groups: (1) *linoleic acid* (LA, or Omega 6); and (2) *alpha-linoleic acid* (LNA, or Omega 3). People who have a degenerative disease such as MS are generally deficient in LNA. Therefore, in the short-term, the intake of LNA must be increased. The best sources of LNA are flax oil and hemp seed oil, as well as fish (although fish is often a food sensitivity source). I took 1,000 mg of flax oil capsules a day (or 2 heaped tablespoons of ground flax seed) at the start of my recovery (if taking the latter, make sure you drink extra water throughout the day). The advantage to taking ground flax seed is that (a) the oil is at its freshest, and (b) it is good roughage for the diet. You can use a coffee grinder to grind your flax seed. Personally, I use ground flax seed in my breakfast smoothie (which I will outline in the Sample Meal Plans section of this handbook), but taking flax oil in capsule form, or indeed straight out of the bottle, is just as effective. Make sure that any flax oil you buy has not been exposed to light, oxygen or heat, which destroy the oil.

At the same time as you increase your LNA, make sure you get enough anti-oxidants. This is very important, as EFAs can encourage the formation of free radicals in the body. In themselves, free radicals are essential to our health, playing a large part in the oxidation reactions, which produce energy for our cells. However, if there are too many of them, they can do damage to our cells, and that is why taking anti-oxidants is important. Make sure you take the anti-oxidants Vitamins C, E and A, plus the minerals manganese, selenium and zinc. Pycnogenol is also a good anti-oxidant.

Although your intake of LNA is the priority, you must also maintain your intake of LA. Major sources of LA are sunflower oil and sunflower seeds, walnuts, pumpkin seeds, hemp and soybeans. For the first 6 months of your immune system repair, it is recommended to try to maintain a 4:1 ratio (i.e. 4 units of LNA for every 1 unit of LA).

However, prolonged intake of such a high ratio of LNA will eventually lead to LA deficiency. Therefore, after 6 months of taking a high amount of LNA, it is recommended to reduce your ratio of LNA:LA to 1:2.5 or 1:3 (i.e. 1 unit of LNA for every 2 ½ or 3 units of LA).

Regarding olive oil, I would like to point out that, although it is a healthy food to eat, it does not contain a particularly high level of

EFAs (about 8-10% LA and about 1% LNA). It is instead rich in *oleic acid*, also found in almond, peanut, pistachio, pecan, rape seed, hazelnut, cashew and macadamia oils. It improves and maintains health, but when you are repairing your immune system, EFAs should be your main concern. Try mixing EFAs with olive oil to make delicious salad dressings.

Evening Primrose Oil

Evening Primrose Oil, an oil which contains 72% LA, also contains 9% *Gamma-Linoleic Acid* (GLA), which has been found to be particularly effective in correcting essential fatty acid blood abnormalities in MS patients. Studies have shown that Evening Primrose Oil effectively causes blood platelets to be less sticky and to speed up the mobility of red blood cells (which generally move slower in people with MS).

Along with cutting out gluten, I consider starting to take Evening Primrose Oil one of the most crucial steps in my recovery. I have continued to take Evening Primrose Oil post-recovery. Initially, I took 1,500 mg three times a day (for a total of 4,500 mg). Seven years later I am still taking 3,000 mg a day.

It is important to take Vitamin E along with Evening Primrose Oil, because Vitamin E is an anti-oxidant that works well with this particular oil. And in order for Evening Primrose Oil to be successfully metabolised by your body, you must also take Vitamins C, B6 and B3 (otherwise known as Niacin), plus Zinc and Magnesium. (Further information is given in Vitamins and Supplements below.)

Hemp Oil

Later in your recovery (i.e. after a year), you might like to try Hemp Oil, which has the perfect balance of LA, LNA and GLA, namely, approximately 57% LA, 19% LNA, and 1.7% GLA. However, personally I could never get to much like the taste of Hemp Oil, even buried in salad dressings, but a lot of people do like it, and if you do, wonderful!

Heated Oils Bad: Unheated Oils Good

When you have a weak immune system and you are trying to repair it, you must not eat heated oils i.e. no frying! Why is this? Because heat changes the molecular structure of oils and damages them, making them toxic to our health. This applies to all oils, but particularly to oils that contain a large amount of EFAs. Personally, I *never* heat oils that contain high amounts of EFAs, such as flax oil, sunflower oil, hemp oil, walnut oil, and canola (or rape seed) oil. Olive oil is a low EFA oil, but preferably should still not be heated while you are in recovery.

You can 'fry' your ingredients in a little shallow water instead, and add your oil to the meal after you've placed it on the plate. This way you can still enjoy that oily texture without heating the oil.

I stuck to this regime for 2 years. After that, I began to use the old Chinese trick of starting off frying by putting water in the frying pan, and then adding a little butter or olive oil to it. This keeps the temperature at no more than 100 degrees Celsius (the temperature at which water boils), and prevents the fat/oil from becoming dangerously heated. As I mentioned above, I *never* heat a high EFA oil.

When you have sufficiently recovered, if you absolutely *must* fry, then use butter or tropical fats, which contain the lowest amounts of EFAs and are least toxic when heated.

Hydrogenated Oils

Oil becomes hydrogenated when hydrogen is added in the presence of a catalyst. Oil manufacturers do this to create products with shelf life (i.e. the oil doesn't go off) and to improve oils' stability at room temperature. Hydrogenated oils also provide what is called the 'mouth factor' in many mass market products, and particularly in the food industry's newest dubious scheme – low-fat products.

You will find hydrogenated oil and partially-hydrogenated oil in products such as potato crisps, margarine, shortening, biscuits, cakes, chocolate, and refined oils used for frying, such as sunflower oil (*not* the healthy kind discussed above!), palm oil and vegetable oil. These are not oils, they are poisons, which contain *trans*-fatty acids. According to the Harvard School of Public Health, *trans*-fatty acids interfere with the body's EFA function, attack the liver, make platelets more sticky, interfere with insulin production and increase cholesterol. It doesn't matter whether the oil began life as a saturated fat (e.g. coconut, palm) or a polyunsaturated fat (e.g. sunflower): the hydrogenation process ruins all.

You might be interested to learn that, as of 2006, the American FDA (Food and Drug Administration) requires specific labelling of *trans*-fatty acids (also known as trans fat) on foods. It took several lawsuits and nearly a decade-long battle between food processors and health groups, but we got there in the end!

Now, as margarine is generally a hydrogenated product, I choose not to eat it. Instead, I eat butter, which is a natural product and much less likely to harm your cholesterol level than a *trans*-fatty acid. I keep the butter down to a minimum though, in keeping with the Swank Diet of no more than 15 grams of saturated fat a day for people with MS.

Hydrogenated Oil in Gluten-Free Products

I would like to especially draw your attention to the vast range of gluten-free products on supermarket (and health shop) shelves that are no doubt going to attract your attention. As mentioned in the Gluten section above, it is wonderful that gluten-intolerance is now recognised and catered for, but why do you think there has been such a rush by manufacturers to get gluten-free biscuits, cakes, breads and other goodies to the shelves? To make money, of course! And one of their best money-making processes is to make sure these products have 'mouth appeal'. Next time you are tempted to buy one of these tasty-looking treats, read the label: I can almost guarantee that it will contain hydrogenated, partially hydrogenated, or hydrolysed something-or-other. Not to mention they're heavy on the sugar. Do not eat them. Go home and make your own. And leave out the sugar too. Chopped dates and pineapple are good sweeteners.

Storing Oils

Make sure your EFA oils (and olive oils) are stored in a cool, dimmed place, as heat, light and oxygen all cause oils to deteriorate. If you are buying an EFA oil from the health food shop, make sure it comes in a darkened bottle, that it has been stored in a cold area, and that it says somewhere on the labelling that it has not been heated past an acceptable temperature (which, for an EFA oil such as sunflower or flax, should generally not be more than 85 degrees Celsius). If you are buying olive oil, buy one that says virgin and cold-pressed.

VITAMINS AND MINERALS

Vitamins and minerals are essential for a healthy immune system. A healthy person should normally be able to get them from a healthy diet, but a person ill with an autoimmune disease is going to need supplements. For people with MS, there is typically a deficiency in B_{12}, B_6 and zinc. In my recovery I immediately set out to redress any deficiency. Immediately after breakfast I would pull out my 'pill bag' and get to work on taking my supplements!

What to Take?

My regime was the following:

What	How Much	Briefly Why
Evening Primrose Oil	1,500 mg, 3 x daily	For EFA (LA) and GLA intake
Flax Oil	1000 mg daily (or 2 tbsp ground flax daily)	For EFA (LNA) intake
Vitamin C	1000 mg, 2 x daily	For anti-oxidant intake
Vitamin E	600 i.u. (International Units) daily – this in addition to any Vitamin E in your Evening Primrose capsules	For anti-oxidant intake
Vitamin B Complex (all the B vitamins in balance)	1 capsule daily. Look for a brand that contains 50 mg of B_6	For healthy nerve function and conversion of EFAs
Vitamin B_6	50 mg once daily (in addition to the B Complex)	For healthy nerve function and conversion of EFAs
Vitamin D	400 i.u. daily	For fat conversion

What	How Much	Briefly Why
Zinc	At least 15 mg, 2 x daily	For absorption of B vitamins and the metabolism of EFAs
Magnesium	50 mg daily	For nerve-muscle functions
Selenium	50 micrograms, 2 x daily	For anti-oxidant intake
Manganese	10 mg, 2 x daily	To counterbalance zinc intake
Lecithin	1000 mg daily	For the brain and myelin sheath
Pycnogenol	3 x 25 mg, 3 x daily	For anti-oxidant intake
Spirulina	½ tspn daily	For Vitamin B_{12} intake

It doesn't matter if you are slightly under or over the amounts recommended, but do make sure you are taking a properly balanced Vitamin B Complex (most retail products will be in suitable amounts, but any health food shop will advise you).

The book I used to gain more in-depth information about vitamins and supplements was Judy Graham's *Multiple Sclerosis*.

Vitamin B_{12}

Judy Graham also suggests Vitamin B_{12} injections. However, my Vitamin B_{12} measurement had come back normal. Also, not everyone has access to Vitamin B_{12} injections. I therefore took Vitamin B_{12} in tablet form. When I started to reintroduce bananas into my diet, I supplemented my breakfast smoothie with Spirulina (made from seaweed), which is extremely high in B_{12} and Beta Carotene. I have stuck with this ever since and would highly recommend it.

By the way, if you've ever been on the Oral Contraceptive Pill, I bet you didn't know that this causes a reduction in your B_6, a vitamin necessary for the absorption of B_{12}, thus potentially leading to a B_{12} deficiency, which can lead to nerve damage.

Pycnogenol

Pycnogenol, though expensive, is a super-antioxidant made from the bark of pine trees. It comes from France and is much stronger than both Vitamin C and Vitamin E. Its unique advantage, however, is that it is claimed to be able to cross the blood-brain barrier, which is exactly what you want in MS, as you want to reduce the inflammation on your CNS, not your joints. At first, the recommended method is to take it at a high level (as listed above) so that it saturates your system, but gradually you can reduce it down. Today, seven years later, I continue to take 25-30 mg daily. I consider Pycnogenol a worthwhile expense.

Vitamin D

Vitamin D is the vitamin whose main source is sunlight. Sunlight on the skin triggers Vitamin D production in the body, which helps the body metabolise fats (a problem area for MS sufferers). Doctors will often tell you to keep out of the sun so you don't get over-hot, which can worsen the fatigue and other symptoms. However, one year into my illness I took a two-week holiday in Antigua. I was very nervous of the sun and humidity, and certainly the humidity did make me feel more tired and I suffered more from 'sticky patches' (areas of numbness) on my legs, back and arms than I would have normally. Nevertheless, I do like the sun (although I have never been one to sunbathe, especially between the hours of 10 a.m. and 4 p.m.), and therefore I was out in the sun a lot, taking care to keep loosely covered during the hot time of the day, wear a hat, and spend adequate time in the shade. However, I have no doubt that I received plenty of direct sunlight onto my body and eyes. Two weeks after returning to Canada from this holiday, I noticed a definite improvement in my symptoms.

Since then, I have read various articles which link Vitamin D deficiency to MS. I would therefore say to you, be cautious of humidity, but not of sunlight. Make sure you get a good amount of sunlight onto your body – the face, hands and arms is enough. Personally, in the spring and summer, I like to get 40 minutes of sitting in the sun, or taking a 20-minute walk twice a day. If I'm going to be out longer than 40 minutes, I then apply a sunscreen *after* I've received the 40 minutes directly onto my skin. If I'm out between 12 and 2 p.m., 10 minutes unprotected sun is enough. Remember, you don't want to cause any skin damage, which will depress your immune system. You want to keep your immune system totally focused on repairing itself, not your sunburn because you've been careless!

In winter and autumn I then take my Vitamin D 400 i.u. supplement (do not take more than 1000 i.u. per day – this can lead to symptoms of toxicity). However, this just can't compete with the real thing – sunlight. I hope you're lucky enough to be able to grab a week or two of winter sun!

Eating Raw

Just as heat destroys the EFAs in oils, so does heat destroy vitamins and minerals in food. Nibbling on nuts and raw vegetables during the day will help feed your immune system.

There is a raw food movement out there that says eating 100% raw is the way to go and will cure any illness. When I was in my recovery I did not know anything about this philosophy, but I did conclude that it was common sense to eat as much fresh and uncooked food as possible, particularly nuts and vegetables. You will find it challenging enough to make the necessary changes in your life without adding the extra burden of completely doing away with cooked food. I think this is something you should consider down the road, but for now snack on raw food, eat lots of salads, and take as many fresh vegetable juices as you like, and you'll be doing fine!

Coral Calcium

I can't remember how I found out about this product, but I took it for about six months approximately one year into my recovery and I felt it brought the final step-up I needed. The best way I can describe it is that I felt stronger inside.

I used the Coral Calcium sachets (like tea bags). All you do is place a sachet in a litre of water (preferably distilled water), leave it there, and the water becomes very alkaline, being enriched with ionic calcium and other trace minerals. When you drink the water, its supposed effect is to balance your body's pH, which encourages detoxification and creates an environment where parasites and bad bacteria cannot exist.

You may see Coral Calcium being sold in capsule form, but I used the sachets. Since then I have seen studies indicating that Coral Calcium sachets allow the calcium to be immediately absorbed into the body without having to be digested. For this reason, if you choose to use this product I would suggest you spend your money on the sachets. I am not sure the sachets are sold in stores – if you search on the internet you will find them.

Food Combining

This system of eating recommends you do not mix animal protein with starch, or different types of protein together, in order to achieve optimal digestion of vitamins and minerals contained in food. It is mentioned in Judy Graham's book and also in several anti-Candida diet books, as well as warranting books on its own. It is known as the Hay Diet in England particularly.

I did do a lot of food combining in the early stages of my recovery, as I believed it was easier on the digestion. However, as I approached a year into my program, I started to eat chicken, organic chicken livers and fish with brown rice (i.e. proteins combined with a starch), although I usually ate these proteins with a lot of spices, such as cumin and turmeric, which break down the protein and aid digestion. I avoided proteins with potatoes for a long time.

As you will see from the Menu Plans at the end of this book, I have followed the principles of food combining in the early stages of recovery and only begin to use a little combining of animal protein and starch in the 6-12 month section (and then only if spices are used, which aid in the breakdown of meat, and if the starch is brown rice). It is up to you after that time whether you start to eat animal proteins and starch together again, but I would recommend it be kept to a small percentage of your diet, even for the long term.

By the way, a perfect meal for correct protein balance is: brown rice, kidney beans (or some other bean) and yoghurt.

Not everything good for your immune system is ingested. There are several other things you can do to aid immune system repair. You might come across more in your reading, but below are details of what I did. Everything can be started immediately.

Food Sensitivity Testing

If you can, get tested for food sensitivities. A good naturopath should be able to arrange this. If you are ingesting substances that either weaken or actually cause harm to your immune system, you are not going to perform well against MS. For example, it is no good eating olives, a healthy food, if your body is sensitive to olives. I did something called Interro testing, which works by testing your body's response to the electromagnetic frequency of the food involved. Now, this might sound flaky, but it seemed to work for me and I used the list of foods it came up with (both good and not so good for my body) to help me decide what my immune system was going to be better off with at the time. It's a good idea to have food sensitivity testing re-done after 6 months, as your body may have recovered sufficiently to be able to handle things that it couldn't earlier – it would be a shame to keep avoiding something when you don't have to.

Physiotherapy

If you are having pain (I had terrible neck pain), see if you can get your doctor to send you to a physiotherapist, or use the sports physiotherapist at your gym if you have one. The sports physiotherapist I saw at the time said he had no knowledge of treating inflammation on the CNS as opposed to muscle and joint injuries, but he did know about neck pain and he was able to give me a set of exercises which brought me much relief.

Exercise

Take up some form of exercise, whatever you can manage. Even if you are having problems with your gait, walk around the house for

5 minutes and build the time up slowly. (I can remember walking up and down the corridors of my apartment building when the weather was really too inclement to go outside!) Ideally, walk outside to get some natural daylight on your eyes (no eyeglasses or contacts). If you are able to do more, do it. Bouncing very gently on a rebounder (no jumping if your coordination or balance is off!) is excellent exercise. Some rebounders have a handrail, which will add to your stability.

If you have access to a gym, get an instructor to show you how to stretch properly and how to lift weights and, if you can, incorporate these into your exercise routine.

NOTE: MS sufferers should never exercise to the point of fatigue, as this depresses the immune system.

Qi Gong

Take up some kind of deep breathing and meditation exercise. Yoga is good, but personally I use Qi Gong (pronounced Chi Gung), which is able to be practised lying, sitting or standing, and for this reason would be helpful to anyone suffering from particularly bad MS symptoms where movement is limited. Tai Chi is a more mobile form of Qi Gong. Deep and slow breathing from the abdomen promotes *Qi* (our life energy) and greatly benefits the immune system.

There are books on Qi Gong (I recommend *Qi Gong for Beginners*, by Stanley D. Wilson, which is clearly illustrated), but it would be even better if you could find a Qi Gong or Tai Chi class to go to.

I have continued to practise Qi Gong and ideally do it outside for 20 minutes a day, to help get my quota of daylight at the same time.

Visualization Techniques

Use visualization techniques to help heal your body using your mind. I am not a fan of the 'battle' visualization technique whereby the body's immune system is imagined to be 'attacking' the illness.

After all, the MS sufferer's problem is that the immune system has gone out of control and is attacking the myelin sheath! My method was to imagine a dam wall with cracks, and my immune system tiny workmen slowly repairing it. Another method is to imagine you are surrounded by a warm, healing light. Any image that helps you see your myelin sheath being healed, and your immune system being welcomed back as a friend not a foe, is fine by me.

The MS Personality Profile

Be aware of the personality profile of MS – yes! one really does exist. Neurological disorders are most likely associated with people who are goal-orientated, like to have order in their lives, do not like to waste a minute, like to keep busy, and who get stressed when these objectives are not met. In short, the Control Freak Syndrome! Bearing this in mind, learn to procrastinate a little – what does it really matter if the housework doesn't get done for a day or two? If you're a fast talker, slow down – your mind is having to race to keep up with your lips! Put your body first and let it rest – completely – so your immune system can start the healing. If necessary, you might have to come to a completely new understanding of what you want from life and what's important. You might even have to 'shed' a few people who don't do your health any good!

A TYPICAL DAY

Even though I've tried to help you get started on the path to recovery quickly, I know it can still be difficult to fit everything together, so I've put together a typical day from early on in my own recovery (i.e. the first 3 months). I appreciate your personal circumstances might be very different from mine (young children, long commute to work etc), but do what you can. For meals see the Sample Meal Plans section.

Morning

- Wake up after enough sleep – at least 8 hours
- Drink the glass of water I've had standing at room temperature all night
- Boil the kettle and make a mug of hot water with a slice of lemon in it
- Find a nice place to do my Qi Gong, either inside, or outside if it's warm enough
- Pull out my exercise mat and do some stretching and my physiotherapy exercises
- Go and have a shower and get dressed
- *½ hour should now have passed since drinking the water*
- Make breakfast, incorporating ground flax seed and/or spirulina
- 10 minutes after eating breakfast, take one capsule of Black Walnut (or other candida-fighting supplement)
- 10 minutes after taking Black Walnut, take one Acidophilus capsule
- 10 minutes later take 1,500 mg of Evening Primrose and 3 x 25 mg Pycnogenol
- Go for a 15-20 walk outside, wearing no eyeglasses or contacts lenses
- Come back, make a cup of taheebo tea (using real taheebo bark, not teabags) and sit down for a 15-20 minute rest
- Take 1000 mg flax oil if not using ground flax seed at breakfast today
- Take 1000 mg Vitamin C

- Take 600 i.u. Vitamin E
- Take B Complex
- Take 50 mg Vitamin B_6 (in addition to the B_6 in the B Complex)
- Take 400 i.u. Vitamin D
- Take 15 mg Zinc
- Take 50 mg Magnesium
- Take 50 micrograms Selenium
- Take 10 mg Manganese
- Take 1000 mg Lecithin

Lunchtime

- Make lunch
- 10 minutes after eating lunch, take one capsule of Black Walnut (or other candida-fighting supplement)
- 10 minutes after taking Black Walnut, take one Acidophilus capsule
- 10 minutes later take 1,500 mg of Evening Primrose and 3 x 25 mg Pycnogenol
- Go for a short lie down. Close your eyes. Do visualization technique. Relax.
- Mid-afternoon, make another cup of taheebo tea
- Later, go for another walk or to the gym, or exercise at home, followed by a 15-20 minute rest

Evening

- Make evening meal
- 10 minutes after eating, take one capsule of Black Walnut (or other candida-fighting supplement)
- 10 minutes after taking Black Walnut, take one Acidophilus capsule
- 10 minutes later take 1,500 mg of Evening Primrose and 3 x 25 mg Pycnogenol
- Go for a short lie down. Close your eyes. Do visualization technique. Relax.

- Make a mug of hot water with a slice of lemon
- Take 1000 mg Vitamin C
- Take 15 mg Zinc
- Take 50 micrograms Selenium
- Take 10 mg Manganese
- Do physiotherapy exercises
- Get to bed no later than 10:30 p.m. and get 8 hours sleep

During the day, drink 8 glasses/mugs of water, either room temperature or hotter. Room temperature water causes less stress on the kidneys than drinking cold water.

SAMPLE MEAL PLANS

The following charts are sample meal plans for a week, to help give you some ideas.

- The first meal plan is for the first 6 weeks of your recovery, where you have to be rigid about reducing Candida. The only fruit allowed is fresh pineapple, avocado and tomato. If you can tolerate this plan for longer than 6 weeks (by extending it up to 12 weeks), then do. I myself did it for 12 weeks.

- The second meal plan is for the next stage of your recovery – 3-6 months. The main food reintroduced into this stage is a wider variety of fruit. However, fruit *juices* would not be allowed – too much sugar.

- The third meal plan is for the next stage of your recovery – 6-12 months.

If you have a juicer, add any amount of fresh vegetable juice recipes into your day. For the early stages of your recovery (1-6 months), do not add any fruit juice.

If you are ever hungry between meals, snack on nuts (not peanuts or cashews, as these can contain mould) or make yourself a fresh vegetable juice.

Where possible, buy organic, especially carrots, meat, poultry and dairy - the carrots because they absorb high amounts of chemicals in the field, and the meat, poultry and dairy because of the high use of antibiotics and growth hormones in animal farming.

Drink two or more cups of taheebo tea a day. In the third stage of my recovery plan (6-12 months), I introduced green tea (leaves, not tea bags) as a welcome change.

From one year onwards, you can try adding other foods back into your diet, but always keep your saturated fat and sugar level low in line with the Swank Diet, and continue taking acidophilus supplements and EFAs. Do not ever eat gluten.

SAMPLE MEAL PLAN: 1-12 WEEKS

Rigid! Food combining principles are in effect. The only fruit allowed is fresh pineapple, avocado and tomato.

MONDAY
- ½ hour before eating anything, drink mug of hot water with slice of lemon
- Breakfast: Millet, with a tablespoon of goat's yoghurt, and ground flax seed
- Mid-morning snack: Veggie sticks (e.g. broccoli, courgette, celery)
- Lunch: Mixed tossed salad (green and red lettuce, rocket, radicchio + green pepper + tomatoes + red onion + cucumber) with hummus and walnuts. Dressing of sunflower oil, lemon juice + oregano
- Afternoon snack: Almonds, pumpkin seeds, walnuts
- Dinner: Red kidney bean curry with brown rice (try brown basmati rice, which has a lovely, nutty flavour). Use cumin, coriander, turmeric and red cayenne pepper in the curry. Do not fry with oil: fry with water.

TUESDAY
- ½ hour before eating anything – hot water with slice of lemon
- Breakfast: Greek yoghurt (sheep's or goat's yoghurt) + walnuts and/or hazelnuts
- Mid-morning snack: Rice cake with almond butter (or other nut butter, except peanut)
- Lunch: Celery + carrot + courgette + broccoli sticks + tomatoes, with hummus
- Afternoon snack: Fresh pineapple
- Dinner: Avocado with walnuts and side salad of tossed green leaves

WEDNESDAY
- ½ hour before eating anything – hot water with slice of lemon

- Breakfast: Millet, with a tablespoon of yoghurt, and ground flax seed
- Mid-morning snack: Fresh pineapple
- Lunch: Mixed tossed salad with mixed bean salad added, marinated in olive oil, sunflower oil and lemon juice, with fresh coriander or parsley
- Afternoon snack: Celery and carrot sticks
- Dinner: Oily fish (e.g. mackerel or sardines) with green side salad and tomatoes

THURSDAY

- ½ hour before eating anything – hot water with slice of lemon
- Breakfast: Greek yoghurt (sheep's or goat's) + walnuts and/or hazelnuts
- Mid-morning snack: Veggie sticks (e.g. broccoli, courgette, celery)
- Lunch: Homemade soup e.g. onions, carrots, celery, lentils, zest of a lemon. Do not start by frying; boil only
- Afternoon snack: Rice cake with almond butter
- Dinner: Chicken with steamed green vegetables

FRIDAY

- ½ hour before eating anything – hot water with slice of lemon
- Breakfast: Millet, with a tablespoon of yoghurt, and ground flax seed
- Mid-morning snack: Nuts and seeds
- Lunch: Mixed tossed salad with mixed bean salad added, marinated in olive oil, sunflower oil and lemon juice, with fresh coriander or parsley
- Afternoon snack: Celery sticks and hummus
- Dinner: Avocado with walnuts and side salad of tossed green leaves

SATURDAY

- ½ hour before eating anything – hot water with slice of lemon
- Breakfast: Fresh pineapple and yoghurt (goat's or sheep's)

- Mid-morning snack: Rice cake with almond butter
- Lunch: Salad Nicoise: iceberg lettuce, steamed green beans, tomatoes, egg, tuna. Dressing of olive oil, sunflower oil and lemon juice. NB: no potatoes
- Afternoon snack: Nuts and seeds
- Dinner: Red kidney bean curry with brown rice and fresh spices. Do not fry with oil: fry with water

SUNDAY

- ½ hour before eating anything – hot water with slice of lemon
- Breakfast: Boiled egg with a little bit of butter
- Mid-morning snack: Nuts and seeds
- Lunch: Steamed fish with steamed veggies
- Afternoon snack: Veggie sticks
- Dinner: Fresh green salad with chopped celery, walnuts, sunflower seeds, with a sunflower oil, lemon juice and goat's yoghurt dressing

EVERY DAY

Drink 8 glasses of room temperature water (or hotter if you prefer)
No caffeine at all
No tea bags of any kind

SAMPLE MEAL PLAN: 3-6 MONTHS

Still pretty rigid! A small amount of fruit is reintroduced, but no fruit juices. Food combining principles still in effect.

MONDAY
- ½ hour before eating anything – hot water with slice of lemon
- Breakfast: Fruit smoothie – any mixture of (bananas, pineapple*, mango, avocado) + goat's or sheep's yoghurt and water + 2 tbspns ground flax seed + 2 tbspns olive oil
- Mid-morning snack: Rice cake with almond butter
- Lunch: Mixed tossed salad (green and red lettuce, rocket, radicchio + green pepper + tomatoes + red onion + cucumber) with walnuts. Dressing of olive oil, sunflower oil, lemon juice + oregano
- Afternoon snack: Celery sticks and hummus
- Dinner: Chicken with steamed green vegetables

TUESDAY
- ½ hour before eating anything – hot water with slice of lemon
- Breakfast: Millet, with a tablespoon of yoghurt, and ground flax seed
- Mid-morning snack: Fresh pineapple
- Lunch: Celery + carrot + courgette + broccoli sticks with hummus
- Afternoon snack: Raw mixed nuts
- Dinner: Avocado with side salad of tossed green leaves with julienne of raw carrots and peppers

WEDNESDAY
- ½ hour before eating anything – hot water with slice of lemon
- Breakfast: Greek yoghurt (sheep's or goat's yoghurt) + walnuts and/or hazelnuts
- Mid-morning snack: Raw mixed nuts

- Lunch: Mixed tossed salad with mixed bean salad added, marinated in olive oil, sunflower oil, lemon juice and fresh coriander or parsley
- Afternoon snack: Almonds, pumpkin seeds, walnuts
- Dinner: Steamed fish with steamed green vegetables

THURSDAY

- ½ hour before eating anything – hot water with slice of lemon
- Breakfast: Fruit smoothie – any mixture of (bananas, pineapple*, mango, avocado) + goat's or sheep's yoghurt and water + 2 tbspns ground flax seed + 2 tbspns olive oil
- Mid-morning snack: Rice cake with almond butter
- Lunch: Waldorf salad of celery, apple, walnuts. Dressing of olive oil, lemon juice, yoghurt
- Afternoon snack: Raw mixed nuts
- Dinner: Red kidney bean curry with brown rice and fresh spices. Do not fry with oil: fry with water.

FRIDAY

- ½ hour before eating anything – hot water with slice of lemon
- Breakfast: Millet, with a tablespoon of yoghurt, and ground flax seed
- Mid-morning snack: Fresh pineapple
- Lunch: Salad Nicoise: iceberg lettuce, steamed green beans, tomatoes, egg, tuna. Dressing of olive oil and lemon juice. NB: still no potatoes!
- Afternoon snack: Celery sticks and hummus
- Dinner: Avocado with walnuts and side salad of tossed green leaves with julienne of raw carrots and peppers

SATURDAY

- ½ hour before eating anything – hot water with slice of lemon
- Breakfast: Greek yoghurt (sheep's or goat's yoghurt) + walnuts and/or hazelnuts
- Mid-morning snack: Rice cake with almond butter

- Lunch: Homemade soup e.g. onions, carrots, celery, lentils, zest of a lemon. Do not start by frying: boil only
- Afternoon snack: Veggie sticks
- Dinner: Mixed tossed salad with walnuts and sunflower seeds. Dressing of olive oil, lemon juice + oregano

SUNDAY
- ½ hour before eating anything – hot water with slice of lemon
- Breakfast: Fruit smoothie – any mixture of (bananas, pineapple, mango, avocado) + goat's or sheep's yoghurt and water + 2 tbspns ground flax seed + 2 tbspns olive oil
- Mid-morning snack: Raw mixed nuts
- Lunch: Steamed fish with steamed green vegetables
- Afternoon snack: Celery sticks and hummus
- Dinner: Waldorf salad of celery, apple, walnuts. Dressing of olive oil, lemon juice, yoghurt

* Use only fresh pineapple, not tinned

EVERY DAY
Drink 8 glasses of room temperature water (or hotter if you prefer)
No caffeine at all
No tea bags of any kind

SAMPLE MEAL PLAN: 6-12 MONTHS

Still lots of raw fruit, vegetables and nuts (but not strawberries yet). A small amount of non-cow's milk cheese reintroduced. A small amount of protein/starch combination reintroduced.

MONDAY
- ½ hour before eating anything – hot water with slice of lemon
- Breakfast: Fruit smoothie – any mixture of (bananas, pineapple*, mango, avocado) + goat's or sheep's yoghurt and water + 2 tbspns ground flax seed + 2 tbspns olive oil
- Mid-morning snack: Rice cake with almond butter
- Lunch: Mixed tossed salad (green and red lettuce, rocket, radicchio + green pepper + tomatoes + red onion + cucumber) with crumbled sheep's feta cheese and walnuts. Dressing of olive oil, lemon juice + oregano
- Afternoon snack: Celery sticks and hummus
- Dinner: Chicken curry with brown basmati rice, using fresh cumin, turmeric, coriander and red cayenne pepper. Do not fry with oil: fry with water.

TUESDAY
- ½ hour before eating anything – hot water with slice of lemon
- Breakfast: Greek yoghurt (sheep's or goat's yoghurt) + walnuts and/or hazelnuts + drizzled with honey
- Mid-morning snack: Apple
- Lunch: Celery + carrot + courgette + broccoli sticks with hummus
- Afternoon snack: Rice cake with almond butter
- Dinner: Avocado with side salad of tossed green leaves with julienne of raw carrots and peppers

WEDNESDAY
- ½ hour before eating anything – hot water with slice of lemon
- Breakfast: Boiled eggs
- Mid-morning snack: Raw mixed nuts – walnuts, almonds, brazil nuts, pumpkin seeds

- Lunch: Mixed tossed salad with mixed bean salad added, marinated in olive oil, sunflower oil, lemon juice and fresh coriander or parsley
- Afternoon snack: Celery sticks and hummus
- Dinner: Steamed fish with steamed green vegetables

THURSDAY
- ½ hour before eating anything – hot water with slice of lemon
- Breakfast: Fruit smoothie – any mixture of (bananas, pineapple, mango, avocado) + goat's or sheep's yoghurt and water + 2 tbspns ground flax seed + 2 tbspns olive oil
- Mid-morning snack: Rice cake with almond butter
- Lunch: Waldorf salad of celery, apple, walnuts. Dressing of olive oil, lemon juice, yoghurt
- Afternoon snack: Apple
- Dinner: Vegetarian chilli with brown rice

FRIDAY
- ½ hour before eating anything – hot water with slice of lemon
- Breakfast: Millet, with a tablespoon of yoghurt, and ground flax seed
- Mid-morning snack: Fresh pineapple
- Lunch: Salad Nicoise: iceberg lettuce, steamed green beans, tomatoes, egg, tuna. This time add a very small amount of potato if you want. Dressing of olive oil and lemon juice
- Afternoon snack: Celery sticks and hummus
- Dinner: Roast chicken breast with steamed green vegetables

SATURDAY
- ½ hour before eating anything – hot water with slice of lemon
- Breakfast: Greek yoghurt (sheep's or goat's yoghurt) + walnuts and/or hazelnuts + drizzled with honey
- Mid-morning snack: Raw mixed nuts – walnuts, almonds, brazil nuts, pumpkin seeds

- Lunch: Mixed tossed salad with mixed bean salad added, marinated in olive oil, sunflower oil, lemon juice and fresh coriander or parsley
- Afternoon snack: Rice cake with almond butter
- Dinner: Baked potato – scoop out potato from skin, mix with yoghurt, a few chives, and sheep's milk feta cheese, and put back in skin to eat

SUNDAY

- ½ hour before eating anything – hot water with slice of lemon
- Breakfast: Raw blackberries, raspberries, black-currants, blueberries (not strawberries) + small topping of Greek yoghurt (goat's or sheep's)
- Mid-morning snack: Raw mixed nuts – walnuts, almonds, brazil nuts, pumpkin seeds
- Lunch: Lamb chop with steamed green vegetables
- Afternoon snack: Fresh pineapple
- Dinner: Salad Nicoise: iceberg lettuce, steamed green beans, tomatoes, egg, tuna, potato. Dressing of olive oil and lemon juice

* Only fresh pineapple, not tinned

EVERY DAY

Drink 8 glasses of room temperature water (or hotter if you prefer)
No caffeine at all
No tea bags of any kind

YOUR CONTINUING HEALTH PLAN

I really hope all the things I did work as well for you as they did for me. As I said, I am now eight years past my one and only episode and, although I have been left with very mild sensory distortion in my left hand, I have continued to improve in my overall health and strength, and in fact would say I am healthier now than at any time in my life. Only if I do not get enough sleep do I start to feel 'off', perhaps feeling more buzziness in my hands or sticky patches in my legs. It is true that receiving a wake-up call over one's health can be a blessing in disguise.

I hope that following the advice in this book (and in your other reading) will help you the way it helped me, but do not stop as soon as you start to feel better. Healthy living is for the rest of your life. Keep Candida in check; make sure you consume enough EFAs; get enough vitamins and minerals; exercise; get enough sleep; avoid gluten; and try not to get stressed.

I hope this book has left you feeling positive about all the things you can do to repair your immune system and to slow down, or even halt, the progression of MS. Things may seem overwhelming at first, but after a while they all become second nature. Just remember that your body needs time to heal, and stick with the plan!

Good luck – and good health!

Louise Docherty
February 2006

A GET-STARTED-FAST BIBLIOGRAPHY

Multiple Sclerosis: A Self-Help Guide to Its Management, Judy Graham

Fats that Heal, Fats that Kill, Udo Erasmus

Food and the Gut Reaction, Elaine Gottschall

The Yeast Connection, William G Crook, MD

Who Killed Candida?, Vicki Glassburn

Your Body is Talking; Are You Listening?, Art Martin

Chi Gong: The Ancient Chinese Way to Health, Paul Dong and Aristide Esser

Qi Gong For Beginners, Stanley D. Wilson, Ph.D

Enzyme Nutrition: The Food Enzyme Concept, Dr Edward Howell

The Sunfood Diet Success System, David Wolfe

Printed in Great Britain
by Amazon